ABOUT BUILDING

MUSCLE STRENGTH

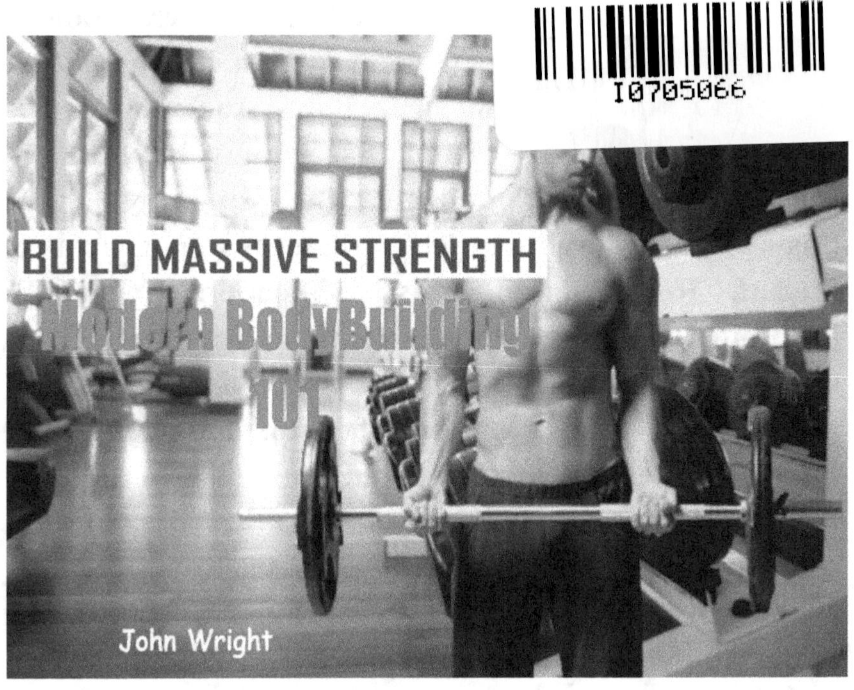

are used are without any consent, and the publication of the trademark is without permission or backing by the trademark owner. All trademarks and brands within this book are for clarifying purposes only and are the owned by the owners themselves, not affiliated with this document.

TABLE OF CONTENTS

NOTES TO THE READER --7

INDEX --8

INTRODUCTION--- 10

CHAPTER 1: HOW TO BUILD MUSCLE FAST - DON'T OVERLOOK THESE MUSCLE BUILDING KEYS ------ 15

CHAPTER 2: ULTIMATE 30 SECOND PULL UP VARIATION ROUTINE BUILDS MASSIVE STRENGTH IN YOUR PULL UP MUSCLES!------------------------------ 19

CHAPTER 3: WORKOUTS GEARED TO BUILD MASSIVE STRENGTH IN YOUR LEGS FOR EXTREME LEG DEVELOPMENT -- 21

CHAPTER 4: 7 EXPLOSIVE EXERCISES TO SHOW YOU HOW TO GET MASSIVE STRENGTH IN YOUR SHOULDERS -- 24

CHAPTER 5: IMPROVING THE DIET AND EXERCISE REGIMEN FOR BUILDING MASSIVE MUSCLE-------- 26

CHAPTER 6: BEST WORKOUT TO GAIN MUSCLE MASS - THE 5 PILARS OF THE PERFECT WEIGHT TRAINING WORKOUT ------------------------------------ 29

CHAPTER 7: 7 EXPLOSIVE EXERCISES TO SHOW YOU HOW TO GET MASSIVE STRENGTH IN YOUR BICEPS --- 32

CHAPTER 8: STRENGTH SECRETS - 3 STEPS TO TAKE TO BUILD SERIOUS STRENGTH! ---------------- 35

CHAPTER 9: HOW TO BUILD BIGGER ARMS FAST - 4 EXERCISES THAT WILL BUILD MASSIVE ARMS ---- 37

CHAPTER 10: HOW TO BUILD MASSIVE MUSCLE WITH CREATINE -- 41

CHAPTER 11: BUILDING MUSCLE - HOW TO BUILD MASSIVE MUSCLE FOR THE HARDGAINER ---------- 43

CHAPTER 12: LOWER BODY TEMPO WORKOUT - THE ONLY WAY TO BUILD MASSIVE MUSCLES ----- 46

CHAPTER 13: BUILDING WITH THE BASIC MOVEMENTS --- 50

CHAPTER 14: STRENGTH TRAINING 101 - HOW TO GET STRONG, BUILD MUSCLE, AND LOSE FAT WITH STRENGTH TRAINING ------------------------------------- 55

CHAPTER 15: EFFECTIVE STRATEGIES FOR YOUR MUSCLE BUILDING DIET AND WORKOUT ------------ 62

CHAPTER 16: 10 REASONS REVEALED WHY YOU ARE NOT BUILDING MUSCLE FAST ---------------------- 65

CHAPTER 17: HOW TO BUILD BIG, MUSCULAR SHOULDERS WITH ISOLATION WORKOUT TECHNIQUES -- 68

CHAPTER 18: MUSCLE BUILDING NITRIC OXIDE - ACHIEVE MASSIVE GAINS ------------------------------------ 71

CHAPTER 19: BODYBUILDING BASICS AND TIPS --- 73

CHAPTER 20: THE BEST WORKOUT ROUTINE TO BUILD MUSCLE - GET RESULTS FAST!------------------- 76

CONCLUSION --- 81

Books by Author --- 84

NOTES TO THE READER

While the authors of this book have made reasonable efforts to ensure the accuracy and timeliness of the information contained herein, the author and publisher assume no liability with respect to loss or damage caused, or alleged to be caused, by any reliance on any information contained herein and disclaim any and all warranties, expressed or implied, as to the accuracy or reliability of said information. The authors make no representations or warranties with respect to the accuracy or completeness of the contents of this work and specifically disclaim all warranties. The advice and strategies contained herein may not be suitable for every situation. It is the complete responsibility of the reader to ensure they are adhering to all local, regional and national laws. This publication is designed to provide accurate and authoritative information in regard to the subject matter covered.

INDEX

Look around. There are countless articles in magazines and online about gaining size and strength. Everyone wants to get strong, and everyone wants to add muscle, but most don't achieve the goal. Why? A number of reasons, including ridiculous exercise selection, poor programming.

If you're willing to do the hard work and make the commitment to using perfect form, this is the ultimate plan for you.

It's a simple plan based on compound movements, high-repetition heavy lifting, and maximum-effort training. Throw in the right assistance work and you've got a plan for success.

Our goals for the next eight weeks are massive increases in strength throughout the whole body, and enhanced muscle size. Don't worry if you don't get super jacked right away. You'll add some muscle now, but the real size will come later on, as you begin to use the newfound strength developed with this program.

Strength is the basis for everything we do in the gym and in life. If you want to get huge, you've got to get strong. Raising your limit strength (the amount you can lift once) allows you to handle a heavier submaximal weight for more reps. Let me illustrate: Generally, low reps build strength and high reps build size, right? Sort of. Well, in this program, you'll be doing a blend of both, but you'll also be doing heavy weights for higher reps.

Using heavy weights for high reps on basic exercises causes a large release of growth hormone in your body and also increases testosterone levels. It's the cheapest growth hormone and testosterone-boosting supplement available.

INTRODUCTION

Building muscle strength is actually pretty easy as long as you have a few key principles down pat. It's a good idea to work on your muscle strength as when you can lift more weight, you cause more muscle fibers to breakdown and thus have the potential to build up more muscle mass. Before we go into how to do it, there's one key distinction we need to make:

Muscle Strength vs. Muscle Size

If building muscle strength is your priority, you will need to put gaining weight to the side. Why? Because the way you approach weight training for strength is fundamentally different from building for mass.

Training For Mass

Let's look at what you need to do to build muscle mass first. If you want size, you're going to need to focus on doing reps with a weight that you can only squeeze out 8-10 reps or so on your first go, this kind of strain on your muscles is optimal for gains in muscle mass rather than muscle strength.

Bodybuilding is the art of modifying the body to appear more muscular and fit. Bodybuilders have to go through a lot of successive training and particular body part oriented weight lifting to get the shape of modern bodybuilders.

Bodybuilding is an art. Anyone at any age can start body building but the quickest gains will come from 18-25 when testosterone levels in men are at their peak. Any beginner bodybuilder will be able to gain muscle quicker than professional body builders or weight lifters because beginners' bodies tend to adapt and respond efficiently to a brand-new stimulus, since they are starting further from their genetic ceiling. The muscles will grow as they will be forced to adapt.

Before starting bodybuilding one must first set his goal and target at sight and motivate himself for being consistent and efficient at every session of workout. Also endurance and patience is the key, the reason being: it takes time to see the muscle build up and grow (you'll notice a difference normally within 1-2 months). Negative thoughts about not be able to build up muscle should strictly be prohibited!

For bodybuilding planning and organizing is of utmost importance. It is not as easy as going to the gym and lifting weights and doing reps and sets. You have to make a routine for the days you will work out and what type of exercises will be performed. It is better to work the counter parts in the same day; if you do sets for chest do the same for back.

The addition of weights on the bar will help to ensure that muscle is properly broken down and can begin to repair and build (muscular hypertrophy), but pushing it too hard at novice level will backfire, so be cautious about it, consult with an expert. Don't work too hard at the beginning; just do one rep short of failure. Total exhaustion should be avoided for beginner bodybuilders.

If you don't have many spare hours in the day, make sure bodybuilding workouts are well planned, and target compound muscle sections.

Finally, rest is essential, not just for beginners, but for all bodybuilders. Without allowing enough recovery time for the muscle tissue to repair itself, you will find that repeating the exercise will cause injury and slow muscle growth. It is also extremely important that your body is provided with the correct nutrients during this time, vegetables are essential, so are BCAAs (Amino Acids) such as Glutamine and Taurine.

Training For Strength

When it comes to training for strength however, staying in the 8-10 rep range for your first set is not going to help you gain much strength. If you want optimal strength gains, you need to look at using a weight which you can just barely get 6 reps out of on the first go.

Once you find this weight, you want to go for those 6 reps, then take a rest and go for 4-5 reps, then take another rest and go for 2-3 reps. This is going to put a lot of stress on your muscles, the type that will lead to massive gains in strength. Later on when you've built up your strength, you can then turn around and do reps of 8-10 to build up size using a heavier weight.

The only other element to building muscle strength is having a good bodybuilding system and diet laid out for you to follow, without a solid plan, many weightlifters fail to reach their full potential.

Here is the Most Stunning Secret You Need to Know to Build Muscle Strength:

If you truly desire to have a ripped physique that gives you a cut above the rest then you definitely need to know how to workout your muscles while building muscle strength. Increasing your muscle strength is not difficult once you know what to do. Below you will find some tips to help you achieve your goal.

Tip #1 - Strength starts with your diet.

You need to supply your body with adequate nutrients so that your muscles can get the fuel it need for growth and repair. Aim to have a balance diet at all times and avoid consuming fried and sugary foods. Have more lean protein and good carbohydrates. You can get your protein from eggs, lean cuts of meat such as beef, pork, and other animal proteins as well as from nuts. For your carbohydrates, you should resort to whole wheat and avoid white flour and refined sugar products.

Tip #2 - Strength training in the gym.

This is very important to building muscle strength. You need to have short intense workouts that are targeted to specific muscles. There is a common misconception that most bodybuilders have that working out long periods in the gym will build muscles faster. The is so far from the truth and will only make you exhausted.

Start lifting light weights and increase as your stamina and confidence builds up. Make sure to stretch your muscles adequately as the only stimulus to make muscles larger and stronger is to stretch them while they contract against resistance.

Tip #3 - Rest your muscles after you workout.

Resting is important to building muscle strength because when you rest your muscle will recuperate from the intense workout and repair damaged tissues. And Anything that helps you recover faster from a hard workout will allow you to do more work to make you stronger.

Follow the tips above and you are well on your way to building lean muscles and increasing your muscle strength.

CHAPTER 1

How To Build Muscle Fast - Don't Overlook These Muscle Building Keys

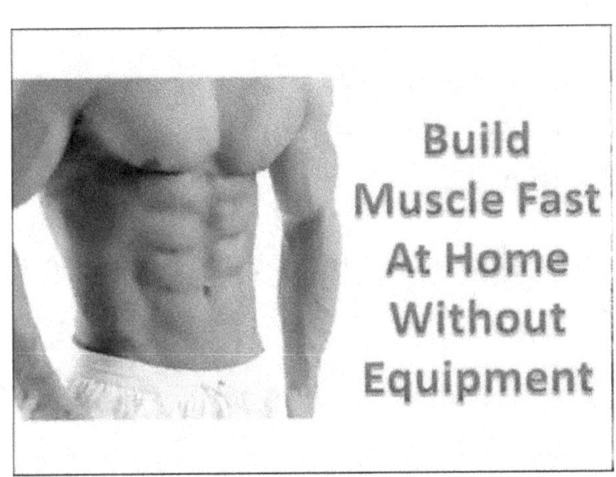

If you're like most guys, you want to learn how to build muscle fast. You've made the decision that you want to work on changing your body and now you are ready to put together an action plan to get to your end goal.

But, you don't want to be left waiting for what seems like months on end to actually see the results happening. No, you want to get results now. You want to go into the gym, put in the work, and start noticing a difference immediately.

There's good news and bad news.

The bad news is that it's unlikely that you will start magically sprouting pounds of new muscle overnight as building muscle is a process in the body, but the good news is that if you utilize the following techniques for how to build muscle fast, you can rest assured that you are going to be well on your way to making the gains you're looking for.

If you work hard and have the right program in place, you could notice marked improvements in as little as two weeks time.

Let's go over the top things to note for how to build muscle fast.

Use Compound Exercises 80% Of The Time

The very first thing that you should be doing is having a good look over your entire workout plan and checking to see which type of exercises dominate it.

Are you doing plenty of bicep curls? Lots of tricep extensions? Are lateral raises crowding out your shoulder workout?

If so, it's time to change that. If you really want to learn how to build muscle fast, you need to think compound.

Compound exercises are the ones that will work the greatest number of muscle fibers at once and will be the movements that stimulate the highest hormonal response, gearing your body up for some serious growth.

Always make sure 80% of all the exercises you're doing are compound in nature. If you do that, you'll be right on track.

Focus On Calories

Second, the next must-do if you want to see results is to focus on your calorie intake. Are you consuming sufficient calories for growth?

Nothing will teach you how to build muscle fast like a high calorie diet will.

If you've been going to the gym for two weeks now and haven't seen the scale budge, that's a very good signal that your diet is causing the problem.

Increase your daily calorie intake by 200-300 and you'll quickly find this problem take care of itself.

Don't Neglect Rest

Moving along, don't forget about rest as well. Remember, your muscles are actually being broken down in the gym. It's after the gym when you rest them that they actually grow back stronger and larger.

Neglect rest and you're really going to short-circuit your results. Remember too that your muscles don't just require rest but your CNS does as well.

You may think you're getting enough rest because you have 48 hours between training any single muscle group, but if you're lifting weights six days a week in the gym, you're continually pounding your CNS.

Eventually, strength will start to decline and you'll see a lack of progress. Aim for no less than two days of rest each and every week. That will be key to getting you results.

Ease Up On Your Cardio Training

Finally, the last thing that you should do is ease up on your cardio training. So many guys think that cardio will help them stay lean while they build muscle but very often cardio is the exact thing that keeps them from learning how to build muscle fast.

If you want to do cardio while building muscle, keep it to once or twice a week and to moderate intensities. Anything more than this will just eat into your progress.

So there you have the top tips for how to build muscle fast. Have a good look at your program and see what might need to be changed.

CHAPTER 2

Ultimate 30 Second Pull Up Variation Routine Builds Massive Strength in Your Pull Up Muscles!

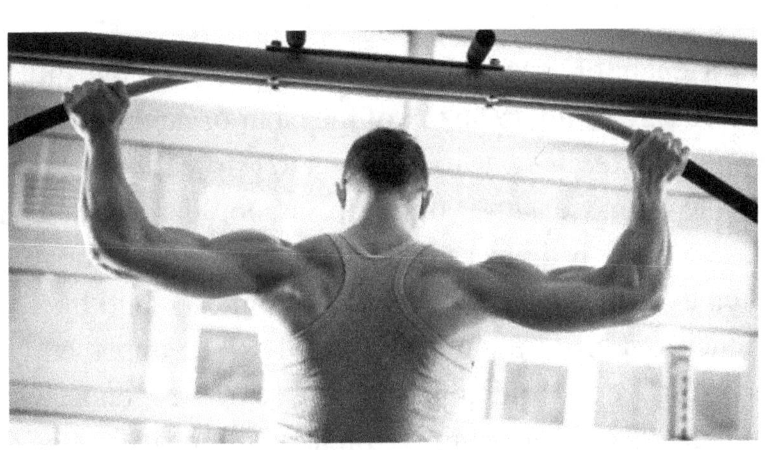

The best way to build, strength and define your back is by doing pull ups. Unfortunately not everyone has the strength right off the bat to be able to do them. This 30 second pull up routine is the best way to build up strength in your pull up muscles. If you do this pull up routine consistently over the following weeks, you will soon be able to do pull up exercises with your entire body weight all on your own!

Pull up exercises are a bit intimidating but you want to be doing them because they are the key to maximum back development. If you are not doing pull up exercises or are not implementing a pull up routine into your weekly workouts, you are really missing out and will not be getting the back results you are looking for!

Here is a 30 second pull up routine that will build your pull up muscles to get you that strength you need to be able to do them with your entire body weight, unassisted, in just a few weeks.

Take a chair or a bench and set it up below the pull up exercise bar. Stand up on top of the chair or bench and grasp the pull up exercise bar in the reverse grip with your palms facing you and ensure your grip is shoulder width apart. Once you are in the set position with your chin above the pull up exercise bar, get a friend or a trainer to pull the chair or bench out from under you so only your upper body is supporting you. Hold this position for 30 seconds. Once complete, take a 1 to 2 minute break and repeat. The goal is to complete 4 sets of this 30 second pull up routine. If you are unable to complete 30 seconds on each set, just do as much as you can and focus on improvement the next time you do this 30 second pull up routine. This exercise should be done ideally at the start of your back work.

This 30 second pull up routine is the best pull up variation to build the strength up to do non assisted pull ups. Until next time, make it a great day planet earth and keep it classy!

CHAPTER 3

Workouts Geared to Build Massive Strength in Your Legs For Extreme Leg Development

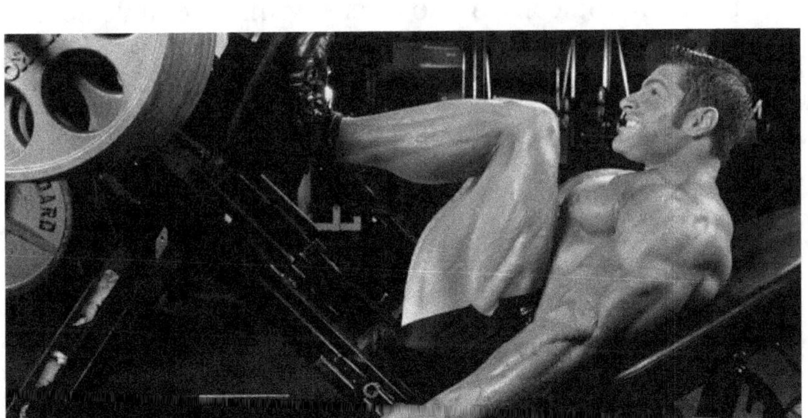

Strength leg development is about combining exercises that demand power and endurance. In order to incorporate both of these aspects into this strength workout, we shall use core leg exercises to improve power and incorporate supersets to aid in improving endurance.

Leg Development Exercise 1: Barbell Back & Front Squats Super Sets

Perform 2 to 4 superset rounds.

Superset Round:

- Back Squats - 10 to 12 Reps
- Superset Immediately with Front Squats - 4 to 8 Reps
- 60 to 90 Second Break
- Front Squats - 10 to 12 Reps
- Superset Immediately with Back Squats - 4 to 8 Reps

Do back squats with a weight you can do 10 to 12 reps with then superset (i.e. no rest between this set) doing front squats with a weight you can do 4 to 8 reps with. Take a 90 second break and then proceed to do front squats with a weight you can do 10 to 12 reps with then superset doing back squats with a weight you can do 4 to 8 reps with. This is equivalent to 1 round. Do 2 to 4 rounds to complete leg development exercise 1. Make sure to use a tempo of 2 seconds up and 2 to 3 seconds down.

Leg Development Exercise 2: Stiff Leg Deadlifts

Perform 4 sets of 10 to 12 reps with 30 to 45 second breaks between sets with a tempo of 2 seconds up and 2 to 3 seconds down.

Leg Development Exercise 3: Smith Machine Lunges

Perform 4 sets of 10 to 12 reps with 30 to 45 second breaks between sets with a tempo of 2 seconds up and 2 to 3 seconds down.

Leg Development Exercise 4: Calf Raise Superset

Perform 3 to 4 superset rounds.

Superset Round:

- Standing Machine Calf Raises - 10 to 20 Reps
- Seated Calf Raises - 10 to 20 Reps

Incorporating this leg development workout into your routine over the coming weeks will help you dramatically increase the strength in your legs!

CHAPTER 4

7 Explosive Exercises to Show You How to Get Massive Strength in Your Shoulders

ow to get massive strength in your shoulders? Use a variety of slow and explosive exercises and move between single set and super sets in order to build bigger, stronger, more defined shoulders with significantly higher muscular endurance.

Incorporate this shoulder workout into your routine over the next 3 to 4 weeks for maximum results.

Exercise 1: Rear Delt Bent Over Cable Raises

2 Sets of Low Weight to Failure for Warm Up. Try and get 20 to 30 reps per set.

Exercise 2: Standing Side Lateral Cable Raises

3 Sets - 8 to 15 Reps

Exercise 3: Slow Front Delt Dumbbell Press

3 Sets - 8 to 12 Reps with a tempo of 2 seconds up and 2 seconds down

Exercise 4: Explosive Rear Delt Bent Over Dumbbell Fly's

3 Sets - 6 to 12 Reps

Exercise 5: Explosive Dumbbell Super Set in Sitting Position - Front Raises, Side Laterals & Bent Over Raises

3 Sets - 6 to 12 Reps per Exercise

Exercise 6: Explosive Barbbell Super Set in Standing Position - Presses & Front Raises

3 Sets - 6 to 12 Reps per Exercise

Exercise 7: Cable Bar Raises

3 Sets - 8 to 10 Reps

As you can see we are moving between non explosive and explosive exercises and moving between single sets and super sets. This is a technique in order to stimulate both the slow twitch and fast twitch muscle fibers and is the best way how to get massive strength in your shoulders.

Implement this shoulder workout into your routine once or twice a week for maximum results.

CHAPTER 5

Improving the Diet and Exercise Regimen for Building Massive Muscle

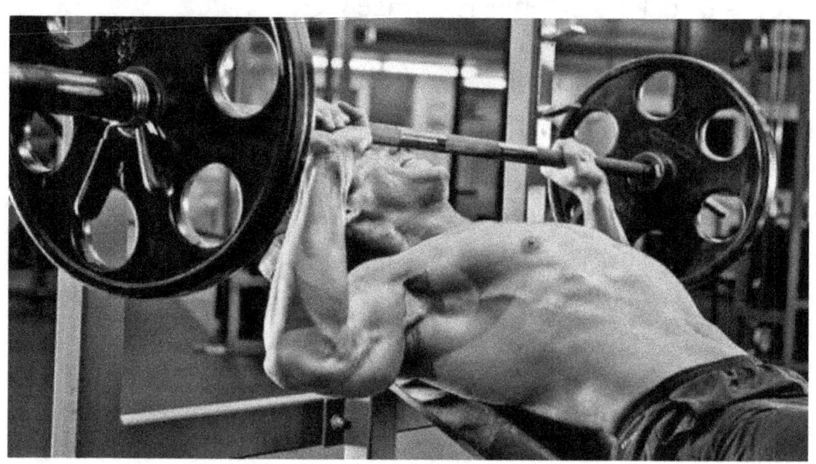

Strength training is an essential part of any successful exercise program; especially for the bodybuilder that is hoping to build muscle mass. Developing muscle mass requires a significant amount of training and dedication, and includes the need to abide by a strict diet and undertake a customized exercise regimen that is much more intense than a standard exercise plan. Whether you are hoping to achieve muscle mass for the aesthetic appeal or competing in bodybuilder competitions, by following a well-planned fitness program including strength and cardiovascular training and a strict diet, the ideal muscle mass is achievable.

Here are some of the steps involved in building muscle:

Diet:

Accepting a healthy and strict diet plan is an essential part of achieving the desired results for building massive muscle. If aiming to build muscle a diet plan is likely to consist of a variety of big, but clean calories. Common foods known to be beneficial for the would-be bodybuilder include healthy fats (fish oil or flax seed), complex carbohydrates, whey protein, turkey, chicken, tuna, a variety of vegetables, and egg whites. Getting professional guidance from a nutritionist is likely to be highly beneficial when it comes to creating the ideal diet program.

Increasing the intake of protein is highly recommended when taking part in a full-time bodybuilding regimen, since it is highly beneficial for repairing and maintaining the connective tissue and muscles. The whey protein shake is likely to help here. You might also want to look at the availability of the supplements like glutamine and creatine, but you should fully research the supplement courses prior to starting on those. A high water intake will also be desirable, with a gallon per day at an ideal level to give the muscles the amount of water required.

Exercise:

Incorporate an exercise program which includes the use of free weights. Free weight exercises are likely to be more difficult when first starting out, but they are able to offer better results for the various muscle groups. A well-planned exercise regimen including the right free weight lifts will result in greater gains by engaging the core and postural muscles more efficiently. A routine including pull ups, seated dips, dead lifts, bench presses, and squats is all likely to help.

A training routine should concentrate on certain muscle groups for each particular workout, and should avoid exercising the same group of muscles for 2 days in a row. A break of 48 to 72 hours is often recommended before exercising the same muscle groups again. And a complete break of 1 or 2 days per week is advised to let the muscles rest and recover.

CHAPTER 6

Best Workout to Gain Muscle Mass - The 5 Pilars of the Perfect Weight Training Workout

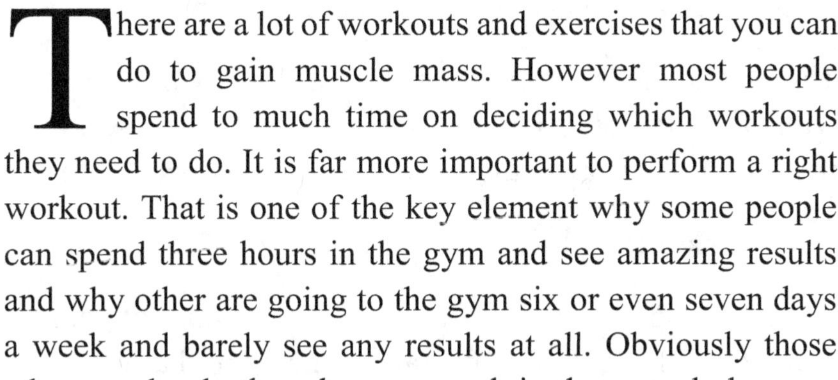

There are a lot of workouts and exercises that you can do to gain muscle mass. However most people spend to much time on deciding which workouts they need to do. It is far more important to perform a right workout. That is one of the key element why some people can spend three hours in the gym and see amazing results and why other are going to the gym six or even seven days a week and barely see any results at all. Obviously those who spend only three hours a week in the gym do have an excellent nutrition programme as well.

1) Muscle treshold

Muscle treshold is simply the amount of work your body achieves in a specific amount of time. Your muscles can only grow when you do give them a reason to grow. To become more muscular you must increase your muscle resistance each and every workout.

2) Activate as many muscle fibers as possible

The next tip to gain muscle mass is to ensure that you have utilized every single muscle fiber within that particular area of the trained muscle. No single muscle fiber can be left untrained or unworked.

To make it clear do not train a few pounds to light.

3) Train with heavy weight for high reps

The workload placed on the muscle is directly proportional with the ability of growing and strengthen your muscles. So perform more work in the same or less time than before.

4) Train to failure

Another important thing to take your muscle gaining workout to the next level is train to the point that you have reached the limit of the muscle. Do not stop your muscle training workout unless you really cannot move the weight anymore.

Taking a set to complete failure is important because it ensures that you have exhausted as many muscle fiber as possible. This is certainly one of the point that the three hours per week guys do and the others not. The guys who are spending (wasting!) to much time in the gym are leaving a lot of precocious muscle fiber untapped and unworked.

5) Measure your intensity

Believe me put these tips into action and you will be amazed about your results. However it is important that your hard workout results in a anabolic environment. Keep track of your process in a training log.

If you are serious about your muscle training workouts and fitness in general then it is recommended to carry a diary. It is important that you have goals for each workout. And the more you have trained the more critical this will be.

CHAPTER 7

7 Explosive Exercises to Show You How to Get Massive Strength in Your Biceps

———•◇•———

So you want to know how to get massive strength in your biceps? The trick is to get creative. The following 7 exercises are unique explosive bicep exercises that you probably typically don't do or haven't heard of before.

Exercise 1: Double Handed Hammer Grip Single Dumbbell Preacher Curl

3 Sets & 8 to 12 Reps per Set

Exercise 2: Isometric Chest & Two Handed Single Dumbbell Preacher Curl

3 Sets & 8 to 12 Reps per Set

Exercise 3: Single Arm Towel Cable Twist Curl

3 Sets & 8 to 12 Reps per Set

Exercise 4: Towel Chin Ups

3 Sets to Failure

Exercise 5: Towel Barbbell Curls

3 Sets & 8 to 10 Reps

Exercise 6: Reverse Barbbell Curls

3 Sets & 8 to 12 Reps per Set

Exercise 7: Free Weight Pinch Curls

3 Sets & 8 to 12 Reps per Set

These exercises obviously put almost all the focus on biceps but throwing in the towel into these exercises enables you to work on your grip strength. Improving your grip strength is key if you want to lift heavier weights in the future and is fundamental on how to get additional strength in your biceps. Equally important is building additional strength in your forearms. Reverse barbell curls get those forearms burning and again are another fundamental on how to get more strength in your biceps.

Do this workout twice a week. Make your first bicep workout a power workout and take 60 to 90 second break between sets. Make your second bicep workout of the week a muscular endurance and conditioning workout. Do the 7 exercises as a circuit and try and take as few breaks as possible between sets. The goal is to be able to complete a circuit with no breaks. Once you have completed the circuit, take a 2 to 3 minute break and repeat. Do 3 circuits to complete the workout.

As you can see, we are really mixing it up and using unconventional explosive exercises that are not typically used. This method of keeping things fresh and new is what keeps your muscles guessing and this s the most important aspect towards further muscle development and is the way on how to get massive strength in your biceps.

CHAPTER 8

Strength Secrets - 3 Steps to Take to Build Serious Strength!

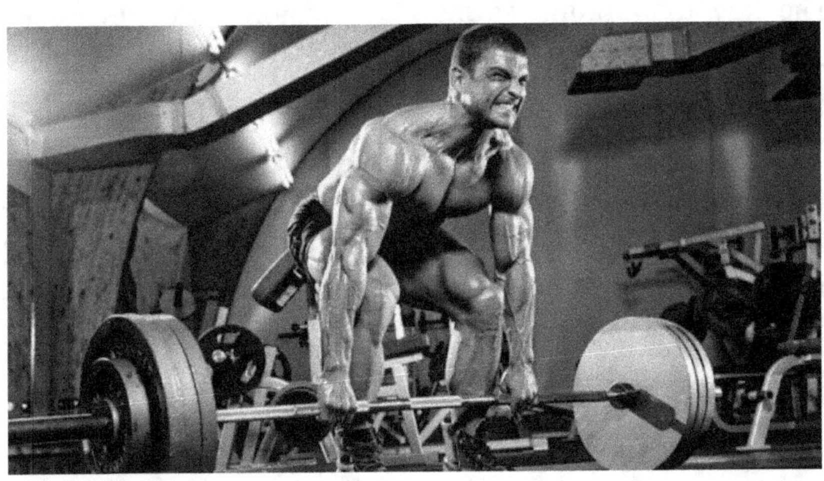

Basic steps here for you to follow in order for you to pack on some real powerful muscle that can produce some real powerful results. Just follow these 3 steps and you will be well on your way to being a true strongman or strong woman!

Step 1: Progressive Overload:

This is a basic principle in the dictionary of building strength. Progressive overload is where you start out with a weight or resistance that you can handle and over time you gradually increase the load to lift heavier and heavier weight. For instance, if you can lift 200 lbs on the deadlift or squat for 5 reps then practice with this weight and then start adding a slight amount of weight each week (like 5 lbs) to bring the weight to 205 and then eventually 210 and so on. You see what happens here!

Step 2: Maximize Tension:

The key to building strength is tension. Strength is the definition of how your body's muscles produce tension. Muscular tension equals force and force equals tension. Maximize tension by engaging in lifting heavier loads more frequently. If we are talking about body-weight exercise and you are great at doing normal push-ups then instead of doing a 100 regular push-ups do 5 one-arm push-ups. Less reps, but more tension! By doing this over time you will develop power. This is why powerlifters are so strong.

Step 3: Multi-Joint Exercise:

This is a definite rule for building muscular power. In order to build massive amounts of strength don't waste a lot of time with those single joint lifts like bicep curls. Instead of doing bicep curls do pull-ups. You don't only train the bicep muscles, but you get your lats, traps, shoulders, and biceps involved in the movement. This is also what stimulates your nervous system and spurs your body's natural production of growth hormone and testosterone! Give it a try.

CHAPTER 9

How to Build Bigger Arms Fast - 4 Exercises That Will Build Massive Arms

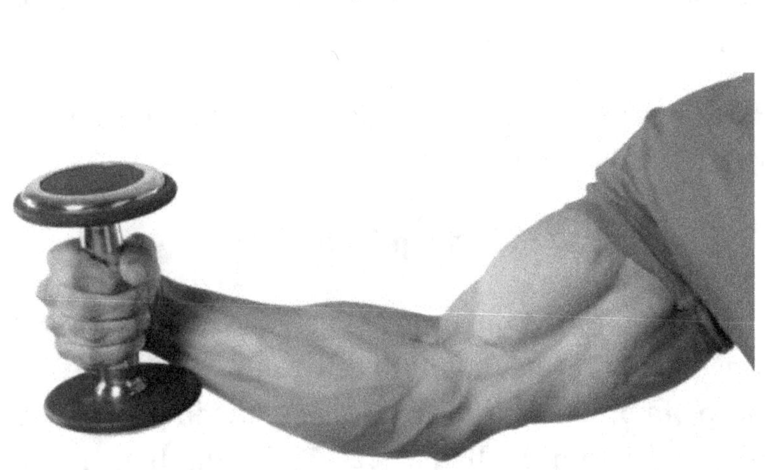

Huge muscular arms are one of the defining points of overall strength. Having arms that stand out can really change the appearance and confidence levels of a person. People day in and day out spend hours in the gym lifting weights in order to try to achieve massive arms, however the sad truth is that most of these people will never achieve a nice set of arms because they are not familiar with what is necessary to build massive arms.

The problem that most people run into is that they put a lot of their focus into training their biceps, when in all reality your biceps are the smallest part of your arms.

In order to know the secret to building big arms you first have to know the anatomy of your arms. The bicep muscle sits on top of the upper arm and makes up about 1/3 of the arm. The tricep sits on the lower portion of the upper arm and makes up about 2/3 of the arm. Then of course there is the forearm muscles which are rarely ever focused on and yet make up the entire lower arm.

Here are 4 exercises you can do on top of your bicep training that will help you to build massive arms.

Tricep Extension

This is one of my favorite tricep exercises because it is a compound movement that really hits all 3 heads of the tricep. In order to perform this exercise simply lay down on the ground with the barbell resting on the floor in front of your head.

Grasp the bar a little less than shoulder width apart and lift it up so that the bar is above your chest. Next without moving your upper arms lower the weight with just your lower arms until the bar is just above your head. Hold for 1 second and then push the weight back up to the starting position.

Close Grip Bench Press

This exercise is again a compound movement that works all three heads of the tricep. In order to perform this exercise all you need to do is set up as if you were going to do a regular bench press. Instead of grabbing the bar shoulder width or greater apart you will now place your hands about 10 inches from each other.

It is important to note that your elbows should be kept as close to your body as possible this will help to really focus on your triceps instead of your chest. Now all you do is perform the motions of a bench press.

Wrist Curl/ Reverse Wrist Curl

Alright now that we have taken care of the upper arm, it is also important that we take care of the lower arm. There is nothing more ridiculous than when a person has huge upper arms and under developed forearms. So to perform the wrist curls all you need to do is sit on a bench or a chair. Take a barbell in your hands and place your hands about 8 inches apart.

Next space your legs out so that the tops of your forearms rest on your legs, and allow your wrists to hang over your knees. Now all you do is simply lower the weight and let it roll down your fingertips and then curl it back up to the starting position.

The reverse wrist curls are the very same deal only instead of holding the weight with an underhand grip you hold it with an overhand grip and instead of resting the tops of your forearms on your legs you would simply rest the bottoms of your forearms on your legs.

CHAPTER 10

How to Build Massive Muscle With Creatine

Taking creatine can really boost your energy during workout. There are a lot of benefits you can get by taking this supplement:

- More energy during workout due to ATP regeneration.
- More power to lift heavier in your workout.
- Less glycolysis which means less lactic acid produced.
- Help you gain weight rapidly given that you have never consumed creatine.

ATP (Adenosine Triphosphate) is the main fuel for muscle contraction. The release of one phosphate from ATP creates extra energy for you to lift weight. By taking creatine, you are supplying your body with more phosphate. This phosphate will then react with ADP and form ATP. The more amount of ATP you have, the more extra energy you can get when you lift weight.

ATP regeneration prevents your body from relying glycolysis, a process that leads to the production of lactic acid. This benefit is clear: the less lactic acid formed enables you to work out longer and harder. You can gain benefits from every repetition you do during workout. You will gain more mass and strength. Another benefit of taking creatine is to keep you from being tired when you lift weight.

The benefits of creatine is not a myth. You can gain significant amount of muscle mass in a short period of time, especially if you have never taken creatine supplement before. It works even better when you stack it with whey protein. During recovery, you supply yourself with enough protein to repair your muscles. Protein is broken down into amino acids which are the building blocks of muscle tissues.

Hard gainers can easily put on some mass with the aid of creatine. The average gain can be ten to twenty pounds in the first month. However, you need to remember that creatine will increase water retention in your body. The gain you make when taking creatine is partly caused by water retention, but the rest of it is pure muscle mass. You'll notice that you are stronger and look more muscular.

Although creatine is naturally produced in the body, the amount is not enough to give any significant effects to your training. Creatine can also be found in fresh meat, fishes, cranberries, etc. Creatine is very sensitive to heat. During cooking preparation, the structure of creatine is most likely be destroyed due to the heat. That is why creatine supplementation is important to give you a boost of power and energy during workout.

CHAPTER 11

Building Muscle - How to Build Massive Muscle For the Hardgainer

Hard gainers often if not always fall into the body type category of ectomorph. People that fall into this category are usually very skinny, and have a small frame. They often have a hard time gaining weight, and can eat almost anything and not gain an ounce. It is often very difficult for these individuals to bulk up, as the more the eat the faster it seems their metabolism goes. It however is not impossible to bulk up, although you will not get all that big, you can still develop an impressive physique.

The biggest thing when trying to bulk as a hard gainer is going to be your nutrition. You have to eat and eat a lot. Just when you think you're full you need to eat another helping. What you need to do is figure out what your daily caloric needs are and then add another 1000-1500 calories on top of that. So if you need 2500 calories a day to maintain you current weight you should be getting about 3500-4000 calories a day. The foods you should be eating are good complex carbohydrates and protein. If you find that you are unable to get this through solid food you can purchase some weight gainer supplementation and some protein powder as well. But the bulk of your daily nutrition should come from solid wholesome foods.

Hard gainers (ectomorphs) when lifting weights should stick to compound exercises such as the bench press, military press, squats, dead-lifts, skull-crushers etc. These exercises focus on more than one muscle group at a time which will induce more growth within the muscle. It is also important to stick to the 6-8 rep range with about 3-4 sets. Every once in a while just to give your muscles a change you can substitute some power sets into your workout, where you stick to the 6-8 rep range 2-3 sets.

Rest is essential as with ectomorphic bodies, your muscles tire very easily and take longer than the other body types to heal. Hard gainers have been known to spend

hours in the gym and usually end up seeing little to no results and in some cases have seen a loss in muscle and strength. Being a hard gainer, when it comes to weight lifting less is more. It is recommended that you only work 1-2 body parts a session and that you get 1-2 days rest in between your workout sessions. Cardio should only be included 2-3 times a week and for no longer than about 30 minutes; as you cannot afford to burn off any extra calories.

Supplementation should include a multivitamin, protein powder, and some oil containing omega 3-6 fatty acids. These will help to replenish your body with the vitamins and minerals that are lost during your workout sessions. This will help to heal your muscles quicker as well.

Gaining weight for hard gainers is never easy and takes a lot of hard work and determination. However if you are consistent with your nutrition, weight lifting sessions, and rest you will definitely start to see results in no time.

CHAPTER 12

Lower Body Tempo Workout - The Only Way to Build Massive Muscles

There is always more than meets the eye when you look closely at all things worth looking at. Take this lower body tempo workout for example. At first glance it looks very basic however I encourage you to give it a go and do it exactly as I have suggested. Be strict with form and timing and you will quickly come to understand that it is not what you do, instead it is how it is done that makes the difference.

The muscles of the body have blood vessels that resemble the root system of a tree. Initially the main root is quite thick and as it spreads further it branches out into finer roots that reach far in search of nutrients. The Arterial system of the human body is very similar with arteries as the main blood vessels that supply the muscles with oxygenated blood and then these branch out in capillaries throughout the entire muscle. At rest blood is pumping through these arteries however only 30% of these arteries are refreshed with new blood with each beat of the heart. The remaining 70% contain blood that is stagnant in movement however full of oxygen in anticipation of movement. Keep this in mind for a moment while you try to understand the following as it is a little deep, so if you do not get it first time then read it again.

When a workout is typically done by most people, the entire muscle is rarely utilized, and instead it is usually the same 30% of fibers that do all the work. When the workout is complete you feel as though you did the best you could however apart from a little pain there is very little growth in endurance, strength, or hypertrophy afterwards. The lack of real progress results in frustration setting in, and the solution is usually to add more weight, however apart from increasing your risk of injury this achieves very little and instead hurts the same 30% of fibers which means the muscle is over trained and tries to protect itself by recovering in a slightly shortened and inflexible state. This the progresses over time into adhesion between surrounding muscles and consequently eventual injury.

Assuming you understand all of that then I will now set out the workout for you to follow, however keep your eyes open for a new video that will be listed in my question and answer section that will address this point in more detail.

The workout consists of 3 exercises for Quadriceps, Hamstrings, and Calves as a warm up and pre fatigue which will slowly but surely saturate the muscles of the lower body with blood in preparation for the final exercise which will overload the muscle entirely to failure. The tempo is two seconds for the lengthening of the muscle, one second at the top and bottom of the movement respectively, and finally one second for the shortening of the muscle.

DO 12 reps, 3 Sets with 60 seconds rest between sets then start the next exercise within 60 seconds.

Exercise 1 is Leg Extension, exercise 2 is Lying Leg Curl, exercise 3 is Donkey Calf Raise.

Within 1 minute of finishing the last set, do 3 sets of 12 reps of Barbell Squats increasing the weight slightly with each set, with 1 minute rest between sets.

Exercise 4a is Barbell Squats with total workout time being 23 minutes.

If you do not have a safe way to do Barbell Squats and want to use Dumbbells instead then you can do as follows. Select a pair of dumbbells that are 85% of the Barbell Squat weight however the tempo changes to 2 seconds down and as fast as possible up. Do 12 reps, rest 10 seconds, do 12, rest 10 seconds, do 12, then you are finished.

Alternative to Barbell Squats is Exercise 4b. Dumbbell Squats. Put a 2cm block under your heels or a 1.25kg weight plate. Should take 2 minutes to complete. Remember to lower you body for two seconds and drive up as fast as possible without rest at the bottom or top. Repeat this 12 times and then rest for 10 seconds whilst simply standing upright and holding the dumbbells. After 10 seconds rest then do another 12 reps. Rest again for 10 seconds then do your final set of 12 reps.

Therefore the total workout time with exercise 4b instead of exercise 4a is is 20 minutes.

CHAPTER 13

Building With The Basic Movements

To get the perspective on mass building we sometimes have to take an outside look at the movements that build massive muscles. To most, building looks like the simplest sport. I must say in the 80's when I started bodybuilding I thought the same idea, of how simple it was that anybody could do this sport. There is no sport that is so very technical like bodybuilding.

Almost everyone in the gym are going nowhere because they do not recognize that bodybuilding is somewhat scientific to a point, it takes more than just lifting heavy weights. While the courage comes from within, knowledge comes from experience. Machine, barbells and dumbbells are just tools that you use, some will work for you and then others will not work so well.

What you do with these tools will simply bring you to the desired results, whether you are training to just have a good physique, contestant or the Olympia you must do specific training. The goal of bodybuilders is to develop muscle mass. Your first step is to lay out a good foundation with barbell movements. You must have a long range view about this and it takes years to build a massive muscular body.

Here are the top exercises that will pack on mountains of muscle on your body:

- Bent-over-rows.
- Bench press.
- Standing Military press.
- Standing barbell curl.
- Squats.
- Standing calf raise.
- Barbell power clean.

These are the seven exercises for building a good foundation that is so important to becoming freaking big. Beginning bodybuilders should master each exercise. Doing cutting exercise is not where mass building is, you will be way off on that note.

These core exercises are the foundation of great bodybuilders because of the neuromuscular activation involved. They are a lot better than machine exercises for building mass because barbell exercises require stabilizing of weights and activate stabilizing muscles which change the nervous system and activate HGH in your body.

Foundation exercise is not as boring as most think, there are many variations to basic movements. Let's take the squat for example; it is not just going up and down. The movement is more complicated. Placement of the bar can change how your thigh responds; small adjustments can prevent injuries like tendinitis. What makes the squat the king of all leg exercises is the neuromuscular activation that we discussed in the beginning of this article. The idea is to master the basic exercises in every possible way.

Regardless of how we are built, the law for mass building applies to all of us. Your DNA has nothing to do with it whether you are an Ectomorph, mesomorph endomorph or ectoplasm. If you train for muscle density rather than muscle mass you will be much more impressive on or off a bodybuilding stage.

Bodybuilding is about balance not height, how they are enhanced depends on the exercise you use. You must select exercises that will allow you to gain mass and thickness all over and give you deep as possible striations.

You should use free weights but do not exclude machines. Free weights bring into play a lot of ancillary muscles and their stabilizers which are not activated with machines and it is these ancillary muscle that fill out your muscles with thickness and balance.

Free weights are motivational, both physically and psychologically. Physically, they demand a do or die attitude. You either complete the exercise movement or you get crushed by the bar loaded with weights. The stress of free weights stimulate internal activity and psychologically of it heightens your awareness that you feel a great sense of pride doing heavy weight by yourself, pushing you even further to see how much you can do.

A myth in bodybuilding is that machines are better than free weight. They are said to allow you to lift with equal balance when really they prevent you from lifting more with one side than with the other, thereby balancing your strength. It is quite the opposite. Machines allow you to push more with one side while the bar stays level. With free weights the weak side must push in order to not lag behind the stronger side.

The result is free weights allow you to bring your lagging body parts into a balance state with the stronger side. Not to say machines are inferior, they have their unique advantages. The only way to reach and isolate some muscles is with machines.

Beginners should use free weights for the first two to three years, to acquaint themselves with the many different free weight exercises there are. Free weights require more work than machines do, so for optimal muscle growth stick with free weights until you have strength and control to the extent you feel confident handling them.

These are the basic universal principles. Your exercises must work the muscles most efficiently. The best exercise is determined by the burn you feel in the muscle you are working. The greater the burn the more mass you will build, so going or feeling the burn should be your goal not doing high reps with less weight or heavy weights for low reps The goal should always be whether for mass or definition, go for the burning feeling, find the best burn for you and stick with it for all sets and watch the size pack on.

Try different mass schedule to see which work for you. Two days on one day off, two days on, two days off or one day on one day off and so on. Start with the muscle group that is hardest for you to build. You choose and always begin with a free weight exercise and go heavy as you can for four to five sets and the other exercises are for shaping. It will defeat the purpose of mass building to go heavy on all exercises.

Your body cannot take an all out heavy set after set as it will go into a depleted state and will slowly grow. Always start with your heaviest sets if you give the first exercise your all. You will have exhausted your reservoir of energy and there will be nothing left for more sets of heavy movements.

By the time you are finished a couple of sets you should be already pumped and can hardly move. So there are seven basic movements that you should never neglect if you want dense mass and that is what these exercise do. Power cleans, bent over rows, bench press, standing military press, squats, barbell curls, standing calf raises.

Years of bodybuilding has validated these exercises as mass builders. If they are performed properly, muscle size is a matter of concentrating on where in the muscle you want that burn to develop or where you want to see mass and it will come.

Muscle grows only when you eat the right foods and get sleep. When you train you break the muscles down therefore try not to train too hard or spend too much time in the gym.

CHAPTER 14

Strength Training 101 - How to Get Strong, Build Muscle, and Lose Fat With Strength Training

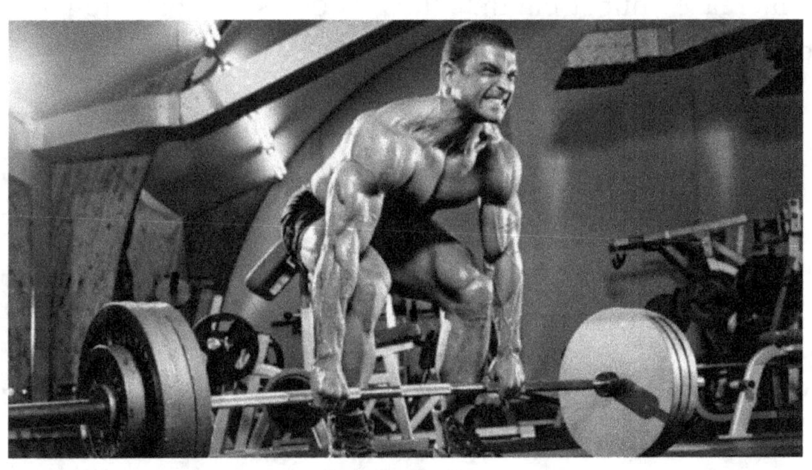

Strength training and physical conditioning is one of the most respected and oldest disciplines around.

The approach is simple. Start where you are and gradually increase your strength. Strength is mainly a SKILL. So like any skill the more you practice it the better you become. Instead of thinking of your strength training days as "workouts" think of them as "practices" instead and you'll make better gains.

Also, strength is mainly a function of your Central Nervous System (CNS). You're basically teaching your central nervous system to contract your muscles harder, in effect "be stronger" to perform at higher and higher levels of strength (as you put them under this pressure through the process of progressive overload). Keep reading to discover more about strength training.

Strength Training - What is it?

Strength training is using exercise and physical conditioning to increase your strength. When it comes to what strength is there are 4 key types:

1) Absolute Strength. This is how much strength you can display irrespective of anything else. Period, bottom line. Strongmen, powerlifters and heavy Olympic lifters are examples of this.

2) Relative Strength. Is being strong, increasing your absolute strength but striving to keep a low bodyweight-basically increasing your strength without increasing your weight. So you are very strong "relative" to how much you weigh. Most athletes would benefit from focusing on this.

3) Speed Strength. Also called "explosive strength" is the type of strength defined by "strength per unit of time" basically how fast or explosively you can display your strength. It's needed in almost every sport and athlete lifters are generally the most explosively strong people around.

4) Strength Endurance. Is the ability to be as strong as possible, as long as possible. You can be strong, but for how long? Can you lift a sub-maximal weight many times? Being able to do high reps on the bench press with your bodyweight... or 500 bodyweight squats is an example of strength endurance, athletes also need this.

Why you Should Strength Train.

Strength training will help you in virtually every area of your life. Here's a partial list of the benefits.

- Muscle Building. Strength training builds muscle - basically your body will grow more muscle to adapt to the demands you place on it through strength training. It's a by-product of increasing your strength.
- Fat Loss. Muscle mass will burn more calories whether you're actively working out, sitting on the couch or sleeping. More muscle mass thus increases your metabolism, which leads to fat loss. Men can get 10% body fat year round (six pack ab levels) by strength training and women can do the same (but at 15-20%).
- Good for your health. You'll not only strengthen your muscles, but also:
  - strengthen your joints
  - get more bone strength
  - Get more endurance and stamina
  - increase your work capacity
  - Increase your testosterone levels

- lower cholesterol and get good blood pressure.
- get better sleep

- Builds Discipline. Strength training builds discipline by teaching you to have a goal and continually work towards it. You achieve success over time-you can use this same principle to achieve anything else in life you want.

Strength Training Methods.

There's different ways to build strength, here's a couple:

- Bodyweight Exercises. Master your own bodyweight first. Pushups, pullups, situps, squats, etc are the best place to start. You move your body around in real life, so it makes sense to get good at moving it around during exercise.

- Weight Training. Using free weights, barbell training specifically. You can build a massive amount of strength, muscle and achieve great fat loss with just a simple Olympic Barbell and weights. Compound exercises like Squats, Deadlifts, Presses, etc build the most strength the fastest.

- Kettlebells. Are a unique way to strength train because they're unique weights. It's basically a heavy weight off-center, it builds "off-balance" strength and is good for your stabilizer muscles this way. Also, you can get just two of these things and work out virtually your whole body (like barbells, they're ideal for home training).

How To Get Started Strength Training.

I recommend first starting with bodyweight exercises and moving on from there to weight training and kettlebell lifting. You need to train your basic movement "patterns" to get strong:

- A Push or Press
- A Pull or Row
- A Squat
- An Explosive Movement preferably involving the hips

That's it. Stick to these basics and you'll do well. You don't need thousands of isolation exercises like you read in bodybuilding magazines. You just need to stick to the basic movement patterns of your body and train yourself to get stronger doing them. Trust me, you'll be using compound exercises which will hit virtually every muscle in your body.

Bodyweight Strength Training.

Pick one of each type of the exercises and perform one set of as many reps as you can till failure to start. Train 5 days a week and two days off. I recommend Monday-Friday and take the weekends off.

- Pushes- Pushups, one-arm pushups, feet-elevated pushups, handstand pushups, etc
- Pulls- Pullups, chinups, horizontal row pullups, etc
- Squats - bodyweight squats, pistols (one-legged squats), deck squats
- Explosive - high jumps onto platforms, jump squats, star jumps, etc...

When you can do 100 pushups, 20 pullups, and 100 squats in the same workout you are ready to start lifting weights. You don't have to do these all non-stop, you could break it up like 20 pushups, 20 squats, 5 pullups, etc until you hit those numbers. Once you can do this workout, you'll be ready to lift weights (and you'll already be looking good and feeling healthy).

Weight Training

Weight training is next. Use a barbell and weights. Here's what to do: Pick one of each type of exercise. Train 3x per week, like Monday, Wednesday, Friday for example and take the rest of the days off. Do 3 sets of 5 reps. Focus on good form first.

- Pushes- Overhead Press, Bench Press, Incline Bench, etc
- Pulls- Weight Pullups & chinups, Bent over Rows, Deadlifts, etc
- Squats - Back squats, Front Squats, Overhead Squats, Deadlift, etc.

- Explosive - Power Clean, High Pulls, Clean and Press, etc...

Here's how you progress: Each weight training session add 5lbs. Do this for 3 sessions in a row, then go back 2 steps. This is called the "3 Steps Forward and Two Steps" back approach to cycling your training. Change up the different types of exercises you do to avoid boredom, but be sure to have one of each type in each training session.

Kettlebell Training:

Kettlebell training is a lot of fun. Pick one of each type of exercise and you can work anywhere from 3-5 days per week. Keep the rep range in the 3-5 and the sets 3-5.

- Pushes- Military Press, one-arm military press, clean and press, bottoms up press, etc
- Pulls- Pullups & Chinups with KB on your feet, High Pulls, Single leg deadlifts, etc
- Squats - Double and single KB Front Squats, Double and single KB Overhead Squats, etc.
- Explosive - Cleans, Snatches, Clean and Jerk, Clean and Press, etc...

Cycle this in the same manner as your weight training. But you'll probably stay with the same weight kettlebell. So you increase the reps. Start with 1 rep and add a rep every session for 3 sessions, then go back two reps on the fourth. The same "3 steps forward, 2 steps" back manner of cycling.

CHAPTER 15

Effective Strategies For Your Muscle Building Diet And Workout

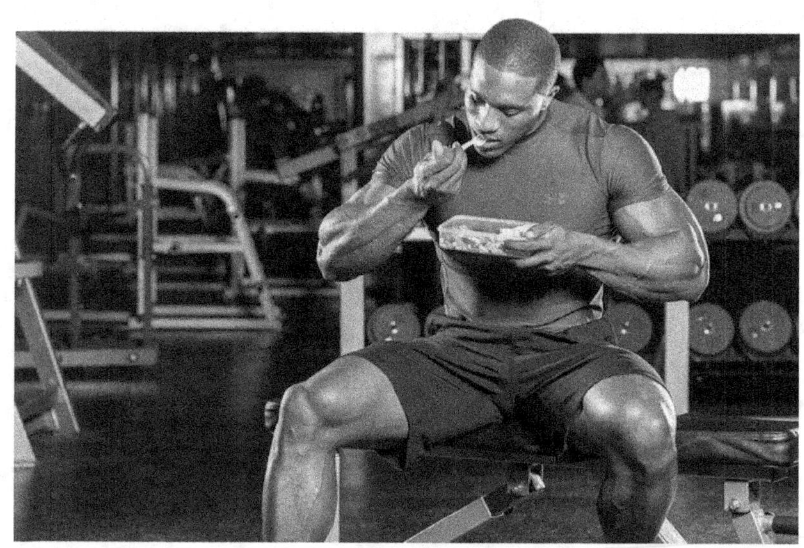

What muscle building diet aids in the bodybuilding machine that your body is? Yes, your body is akin to a machine that reinvents itself constantly. Every minute that ticks during your everyday activity, your body breaks down its tissues and then replaces them with new tissues. This mechanism is fueled by the combination of the foods that you eat. What about when you're building muscles? Your muscle building workouts actually result to muscular break down and muscular build up. Your exercises make this process go faster than it would under normal circumstances. When you're building muscles, a protein takeover mechanism takes place. What makes it more effective in building muscles is when you end up with more muscles than what you started with. How do you make your muscle building workout and diet effective?

You have to be mindful of your muscle building diet to begin with. Eat more proteins than you normally do. Protein, as an anabolic component would like to have itself stored in your muscles. Combine your muscle building diet with a complementary workout routine for building muscles. Your exercises should be able to stress your muscles so that they become stronger and bigger. The power combo of effective muscle building is therefore a super diet of high quality protein along with a massive strength training workout routine. This process is it when you're looking for the oldest and the best non-pharmaceutical technique of building muscles.

How much protein should you eat to build muscles?

During the first 20 days of strength training, the size of your muscles increases by 0.2 percent everyday. This figure is over and above the normal rate of muscle mass growth. If you're just starting out in your program, you'll basically need a heftier amount of protein in your diet than a muscle builder who's been training for years. As a beginner, you thus have to worry more about getting more protein in your muscle building diet.

How much protein do you exactly need? That's.73 gram per pound of your body weight in a day. So if you weigh 180 pounds, your protein needs amounts to 130 grams per day.

How often do you need to eat protein?

Protein synthesis, the process of taking protein from food and converting it into muscles takes place when your body has consumed 20 to 25 grams of high-quality protein. The more protein you take in, the better protein synthesis works. You need to supply more proteins in your muscle building diet. Four hours after your workout, protein synthesis peaks. In this case, you have to eat protein immediately before and after your strength training workout.

Protein supplements make a difference, too. Taking protein supplements makes you gain an additional 2 pounds of muscles in a period of 12 weeks. Experienced muscle builders in fact take pre and post workout protein supplements to achieve maximum strength training results. Take a protein-rich meal 2-3 hours before you train and another of the same meal 1 to 2 hours after you've worked out.

Grow stronger and bigger muscles faster by combining effective techniques in strength training and your muscle building diet.

CHAPTER 16

10 Reasons Revealed Why You Are Not Building Muscle Fast

Most of the time, people who are into building muscle, put a premium on their actual workout routine, but they tend to miss out another important element of building big muscle. Building massive muscle is a process which entails proper nutrition and a structured workout routine. What people forget when building lean muscle is "what to do after following an intensive muscle building routine"? You must adhere to these "Top 10 Secrets to Building Massive Muscle", if you are looking to get rid of your Flabby Muscles:

- First, you're probably not keeping track of what you eat. Find a nutritionist assist to you with this issue, and then you should try to follow what your nutritionist says to the "T".

- Also, it could be possible that even if you are doing rigid training, you have a protein deficient diet which is much less that what your body really needs. Protein is the most essential nutrient in building massive muscles.

- In relation to item number 2, your poor diet can also be a major factor. If you don't have the calories your body requires, you will end up burning more muscle than building huge muscles.

- Additionally, you may be training to the point that your body and muscles don't have adequate amount to rest. Your muscles need some down time to regenerate themselves.

- For another reason, you're training more often than what is required. Overdoing cardiovascular activities everyday won't help build muscle quicker.

- Next, your body might have reached its limitations in regards of strength. It could be a possibility that your body can't handle your intense workouts anymore. Your body may need additional nutrition in order for you to continue building bigger muscle.

- Similarly, you may also be doing more sets than what was recommended by your trainer. The key to building muscle quickly is to carry the proper load, following the right form and doing the appropriate number of sets.

- In addition, you may be working out hard enough or just doing the exercises the wrong way. For your muscles to develop properly, you have to make sure that your form and posture are correct, to work out your muscles to their potential.

- On the contrary, you may have been too relaxed in your training, instead of being very progressive in your weight training.

Lastly, you may not be properly motivated after all. You started off with your work out even though you had no clue on what to do, what you expected of yourself, or what you wanted your body to look. A properly planned goal serves as a helpful guide to build huge muscles fast.

CHAPTER 17

How To Build Big, Muscular Shoulders With Isolation Workout Techniques

When you're out in a muscle tee or tank top, your arms aren't the only body part on display. To look your best, you need well developed shoulders to top off your biceps and triceps. Isolation shoulder training is designed to force the targeted muscle, in this case your deltoids, to perform with minimal assistance from other muscle groups. Seated military presses and dumbbell presses are examples of isolation exercises that, when performed correctly, are very effective for building big, muscular delts.

On the other hand, compound exercises encourage simultaneous and coordinated work between various muscle groups. For example, deadlifts and Olympic lifts like the snatch and clean and jerk illustrate compound weightlifting movements that enlist some power from the shoulders. While these compound movements excel for sport specific conditioning and building overall body strength, isolation training will stimulate maximum growth of the deltoid area.

For example, I recommend seated front and rear military presses for adding mass to the anterior and medial heads of the deltoids. Though these exercises are very effective when done properly, beginning bodybuilders wasting valuable gym time doing them incorrectly. The most common mistake with seated military and/or dumbbell presses is jerking the weight overhead by arching the back or raising the hips from the seat. The whole point of sitting with lower back support to do these exercises is to force the shoulders - namely the anterior and medial deltoids - to power the weight upward without help from the rest of the body. Raising the hips and arching the back not only risks hyperextension of the spine or other injury, but it also defeats the exercise's intended effect.

Seated military and dumbbell presses are designed to build massive delts by isolating resistance on these muscles as much as possible with strict training technique. Such technique requires the controlled pressing of the weight overhead with your butt planted firmly on the seat and your lower back pressed safely against a chair back. Jerking the weight overhead with bodyweight assistance deprives the delts of the work they need to grow and simply wastes time.

While no one would purposely waste time with ineffective workouts, many beginning bodybuilders just don't know how to properly perform isolation training for their delts. Additionally, such beginners are notoriously impatient and they often don't understand that building a truly awesome physique is a process, not an event. As a result, too many beginners start out working with poundage that is too heavy to handle without cheating on training technique.

It's true that progressively increasing your weight resistance in the military and dumbbell presses is essential to building big, muscular delts. But you shouldn't try to work with more weight than you can lift naturally and with proper training technique. Remember, you're not in competition with anyone besides yourself when it comes to maximizing your bodybuilding potential. And the only person who loses if you cheat on your isolation training technique is you! So don't worry about impressing or keeping up with anybody else - especially if you're just starting out. Use safe amounts of weight with proper technique and you'll soon build the big, muscular shoulders that you deserve.

CHAPTER 18

Muscle Building Nitric Oxide - Achieve Massive Gains

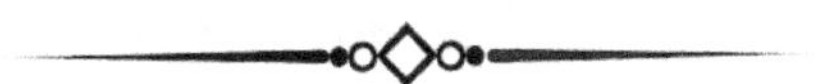

Today there are thousands of supplements on the market. Most of them are not worth the package that they are in. There is one product which is the muscle building nitric oxide that is actually helping people achieve massive gains. This product has been around for a few years and has grown into one of the best sellers. There are many different companies that sell this product or a version of the product.

There are many benefits to the muscle building nitric oxide. This product is known as a vasodilator. This means that it increases blood flow by widening the blood vessels. If this sounds unsafe do not worry because it is 100% safe. The key benefit to doing this is that your muscles will receive more blood during the workout which will allow you to get a better workout. Also most people are excited about the huge muscle pumps you get while on this product.

Some people are noticing as high as a 20% increase in strength because of this supplement. This strength gain is translating to people achieving massive gains in size. Another side benefit to this product is that your recovery times are cut down dramatically. After you workout and drink your protein or eat your meal some magic begins. Since you blood vessels are still enlarged this allows more nutrients to get directly to the muscle. This allows them to repair and grow faster.

The muscle building nitric oxide is the go to supplement for many of today's bodybuilders and serious weightlifters. You too can start achieving massive gains by using this product. It is 100% safe and effective so why not give it a try, you will not be sorry.

CHAPTER 19

Bodybuilding Basics and Tips

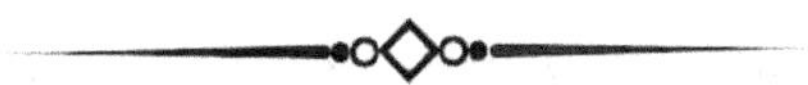

Ever since the first pre-human picked up a heavy rock a number of times and found his muscles pumped, mankind has been into bodybuilding. The first efforts were to refine and define the musculature needed to throw a spear farther, or pull a stronger bowstring, or thrust a sword harder. Later efforts involved athletic contests, with very specific bodybuilding training for the muscles needed for wrestling, running, jumping and other sports. In modern times, bodybuilding has evolved into an end unto itself, with a conditioned, sculptured, all-over musculature being the primary purpose.

Bodybuilding basics should begin with an established goal. What is the purpose of the exercise? Most beginners start with a modest goal of getting fit, losing the "middle-aged spread," but as they start seeing results, they raise the bar of their expectations... and they will see and feel results after a surprisingly brief period of time. If the goal is the loss of a set amount of weight, the beginner will not see a weight loss as quickly as they see visual results because as the muscles develop they increase in density and weight, even though certain body parts appear smaller. Weight loss is not a particularly good initial goal because of this, but may be a good longer term goal.

Most bodybuilding basics involve weight training in some form; free-weights (barbells, dumbbells, kettle bells); machines (Nautilus, HammerStrength, etc.), or bodyweight exercises (push-ups, pull-ups, jumping-jacks, lunges). The resistance of the weights, used in multiple sets of multiple repetitions, causes a breakdown in the muscle tissue, which when it rebuilds, is larger and stronger. Theoretically, the more weight used coupled with the more often it is used, the bigger and quicker the results, at least this was the early hypothesis. Modern bodybuilding is a combination of the proper approach to the exercises, coupled with a nutritional diet and plenty of rest.

A beginning bodybuilder should seek professional advice at their fitness center of choice. A good personal trainer will develop a program of bodybuilding basics specifically tailored to the beginner's needs, one of a good combination of interval training with weights for the entire body, cardio-vascular exercises for the heart and lungs and good nutritional suggestions. If a fitness center isn't available, it would be best to start with bodyweight resistance exercises. Running and bodyweight squats and lunges will take care of the lower body and cardio. The following are for the upper body.

- Push-ups - on the floor, prone with hands placed at shoulder width, push the body off the floor while rising on the toes. Ten repetitions, one minute rest, repeat, rest, repeat. If unable to complete ten reps, keep knees on floor lessening the resistance. Do them this way until able to complete fifteen or twenty reps, and then go to full push-ups. As conditioning improves, elevate the feet to increase resistance.

- Pull-ups or Chins - rig a bar in a doorway or make a pull-up bar from ¾ inch pipe and hang it over a rafter in the garage. Begin with hands at shoulder width, palms forward, grasp the bar and let your body hang full length, bending you knees if the bar is too close to the floor to all a full length hang. Pull yourself up until you chin is over the bar, let yourself back down slowly, then repeat nine more times. If unable to do more than a few pull-ups, position a chair so that you may bend your knees and hook your toes over the edge of the chair to lessen the weight resistance.

- Bicep Pull-ups - using the same bar, reverse your palms so that when you pull-up the bicep is being used more, rather than the back and shoulders as in the regular pull-up.

- Triceps Press - Position two chairs far enough apart so that feet may be placed on one and the hands on the other while in a supine position. Lower the body to the floor, or until the triceps are fully extended, push you body back up, repeat nine more times.

CHAPTER 20

The Best Workout Routine to Build Muscle - Get Results Fast!

—•◇•—

Ask almost any bodybuilder, powerlifter, or other big, strong dude, and he'll tell you there's no one way to train for building muscle and strength. Even so, you constantly get guys asking you "what's the best workout routine to build muscle?" "What's the one way to train that will really get me the best results?"

Truth is, most of these guys aren't really looking to learn any valuable information or put in any serious work at the gym. They're looking for a magic bullet, that "secret" workout that will get them a big chest, strong arms, and washboard abs by yesterday. That's not going to happen!

But then again, you're not that kind of trainee, are you? You really do want to know exactly how to build muscle, and you're willing to put in the work to make it happen. You just want to know what the best workout routine to build muscle is so that you can maximize the time you put in at the gym! Truth be told, there is no single, best routine, but there are a few rules you MUST follow to make quick progress. Tailor your training to these principles, and you WILL get bigger and stronger faster than you ever thought possible...

1. Squatting for Size

Many an old-timer, washed-up meathead will tell you that squats are the king of all exercises. Don't ignore them just because they aren't in their prime, they're right! Squats are truly the best overall mass-building exercise you can do, but they have unfortunately gone by the wayside as companies have developed new and fancy leg press and hack squat machines. Those have their place too, but they will NEVER replace the good ol' squat.

You can spend years perfecting your squat technique and routine, but here are a few tips that will put you head and shoulders above 99% of the other gym rats. First, take a medium-width stance, slightly wider than your shoulders. Don't buy into that "close stance to work the quads" crap, your quads will get bigger as long as you squat big weights.

Next, place the bar low on your upper back, pinching your shoulder blades back as tight as possible to create a "shelf" for the bar with your shoulders. Take the bar out of the rack in a controlled but firm manner, KNOWING you're going to dominate that weight. Once you've taken a couple steps back, fill your belly with air (not your chest!), and sit BACK and down into the squat.

That backwards motion with your hips is essential for bringing your hamstrings and glutes into the equation and allowing you to lift some serious weight. You'll never squat big if you just worry about your quads! Once the crease of your hip is at the same level as your knees (this is called parallel), explode back up to the starting position.

As far as actual routines go, there are tons of ways to train the squat. For a beginner or intermediate, I would recommend a routine where you've got one "lower body" or "legs" day where you focus on squatting as your primary exercise, working up to one or two heavy sets of 4-6 reps. You should strive to increase the weight on these sets week after week. Follow up your squatting with other leg exercises like lunges and leg presses, and you're good to go. Remember, your legs have as much or more muscle mass than your entire upper body, so get them big!

2. Strength? Size? It's all the Same!

If you read any conventional bodybuilding "wisdom" these days, you'll see most guys talking as if size and strength are two totally different goals, and that you have to focus on one or the other. What a bunch of crap! Stereotypes of the "all show and no go" bodybuilder aside, have you really ever seen someone who was massively muscular and NOT strong? No way!

The thing is, your muscles grow in response to certain stimuli. There are a number of ways to stimulate this growth, but the only one that can work in the long term is getting stronger. Think about it, if you increase your bench by 100 pounds, do you think you'll have bigger pecs? If you take your max on the squat and get strong enough to rep it 10 times, do you think your legs will be bigger? Of course!

Traditional bodybuilding split, powerlifting workout, 5 x 5, it all works. The thing that really matters is that you get stronger! If you train your heart out but don't worry about actually getting stronger, I guarantee that you will be the same size as you are now, six months or a year from now. Now THAT is wasted time.

There are tons and tons of ways to go about getting stronger, but the main thing you should worry about is gradually adding weight to the bar, week after week, for sets of 4-6 reps. Fewer or more reps is alright if you really want to, but the important thing is to always focus on the weight. Don't get too eager, either. A five pound increase per week on the squat or bench may seem like next to nothing, but if you did that for a few months, you'd have made over a 100 pound increase in your strength!

3. Massive Food for Massive Gains

Hopefully you already know this, but just in case it's not drilled into your head yet, I'll say it again - nutrition is THE most important aspect of bodybuilding. You can have the perfect routine and stick to it like a champion, but at the end of the day, your body still needs enough nutrients to repair damage muscle tissue and build it bigger than it was before.

Proper bodybuilding nutrition is actually somewhat well-known these days, so I'll just give you the quick and dirty on how to eat for lean muscle gains. First, you want tons of protein. If you get one gram of protein per pound of your own bodyweight per day (not counting the incidental amounts in grains), then you're on the right track.

Second, you've got to get extra calories from fats and carbs to have the energy to train and grow. Don't bother getting out calculator or counting calories, though. Just make sure you eat most of your carbs before and after training and eat fats with your proteins during the rest of the day. For carbs, eat nutritious foods like oats, other grains, and potatoes. For fats, take in plenty of olive oil, nuts, avocados, and some red meat.

CONCLUSION

If you want to build the kind of strength that will intimidate and impress, then you need look no further than the world of bodybuilding. This is a community and discipline that is filled with gigantic beasts of men, most of whom are all-too happy to share their secrets when it comes to disclosing precisely how they built such a massive amount of strength and power.

And largely what these secrets consist of is techniques that can be used to help make workouts more intense such that more microtears are created in the muscles leading to more subsequent growth and strength gains.

Some of these techniques are better known than others though, and one of the most powerful but lesser-known is the incredible 'mechanical drop set'.

Bodybuilding is a sport that requires a huge amount of discipline on the part of the bodybuilder. In fact, discipline is what drives any good training program. That is because discipline brings about consistency on the manner on how any bodybuilder trains and handles his or her workout program. Disciplined bodybuilders do not waver in their workout regimen or merely go through the motions. Whether rain or shine, tired or full of energy, disciplined bodybuilders are able to make sure that they watch their diet and supplement intake everyday and devote a certain amount of time to workout in the gym.

There are a number of other factors that can spell success or disaster into one's training program. Here are just a few bodybuilding tips and tricks that are guaranteed to help any bodybuilder achieve his or her goals for this New Year.

It is important for every bodybuilder to ensure that his or her body gets just the right nutrients not only to stay healthy, but to help it get the cuts and build the muscle mass one envisions to achieve. Even beginners to bodybuilding or any fitness training program for that matter understands that protein is one of the most important nutritional supplements to consume. But it is not just the only nutrient that is essential for every bodybuilder. Multi-vitamins are just as important as proteins, but they are also the most underestimated supplements that a bodybuilder can consume. Multi-vitamin supplements help ensure that bodybuilders get all the vitamins and minerals they need for hardcore training, growth and health.

Thank you again for downloading this book!

I hope this book was able to help you to gain your true happiness, via positive thinking always. Life is way to short to mope along, enjoy the time you have been given and the blessings you have. The next step is to actually practice each technique until it becomes a habit. Reading alone will do nothing for you. Please be proactive with your fitness and positive mindset.

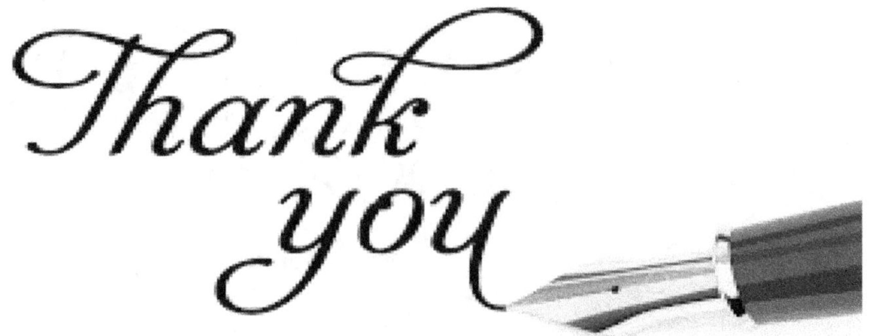

Finally, I hope this book has brought you much joy as it has for me. I'd like to ask you for a favor, would you be kind enough to leave a review for this book on Amazon? It'd be greatly appreciated!

Books by Author

Please feel free to browse through our selection of other books.

Thank you and good luck!

3 Day Detox Green Smoothie Cleanse

https://www.amazon.com/Green-Smoothie-Cleanse-Metabolism-Smoothies-ebook/dp/B06WVV56XJ

How To Build Muscle And Burn Fat For Women

https://www.amazon.com/Build-Muscle-Burn-Fat-Stronger-ebook/dp/B06WWQQ4MZ

The Ketogenic Diet - Burn Up To 1 Pound Per Day In Ketosis

https://www.amazon.com/dp/B06XFWHL2W/ref=sr_1_21?s=digital-text&ie=UTF8&qid=1488906467&sr=1-21&keywords=ketogenic+diet

10 Minute Abs...Invest 10 Minutes Per Day Achieve A Flatter Belly Feel Lean For Life (Abs, Abs Workout, Abs Diet, Abs Training, Shredded Abs, Flat Belly, Flat Belly Diet)

https://www.amazon.com/Abs-Minutes-Achieve-Training-Shredded-ebook/dp/B06XRTSYQK

Build Massive Strength... Modern BodyBuilding 101 (Build Muscle, Lean Muscle Mass, Weight Training, Bodybuilding Nutrition, Build Muscle Fast, Thinner, Leaner, Stronger) https://www.amazon.com/dp/B06XV6RK3R

How To Build Muscle And Burn Fat For MEN…Lean For Life! (Build Muscle Lose Fat, Lean Muscle Diet, Fitness Books, bodybuilding for … Build Muscle Fast, Thinner, Leaner)

https://www.amazon.com/dp/B06XVVW6HP

*Meal Prep…Abs Are Made In The F*cking Kitchen (Meal Prep, Meal Prepping, Nutrition Facts, Deep Nutrition)*

https://www.amazon.com/dp/B06XW25DZ9